Human Reproduction
Basic Anatomy and Physiology

Akmal El-Mazny

Copyright © 2014 Akmal El-Mazny

All rights reserved.

CreateSpace, Charleston SC, USA

ISBN-13: 978-1494492816
ISBN-10: 1494492814

Contents

Introduction	1
MALE REPRODUCTIVE SYSTEM	
Overview	2
Testes	5
– Hormonal Control	11
– Spermatogenesis	13
Duct System	18
Accessory Glands	25
Penis	31
– Erection and Ejaculation	34
FEMALE REPRODUCTIVE SYSTEM	
Overview	36
Ovaries	37
– Hormonal Control	40
– Ovarian Cycle	48
– Oocyte Development	53
Uterine Tubes	57
– Fertilization	59
Uterus	61
– Menstrual Cycle	64
– Implantation	67
– Embryo Development	68
Cervix	72
Vagina	74
External Genitalia	76
References	80

INTRODUCTION

The male and female reproductive systems consist of the gonads, testes or ovaries; the reproductive tract; the external genitalia; and the hypothalamic-pituitary unit.

The functions of the reproductive system are to produce and deliver gametes, spermatozoa or oocytes, for sexual reproduction; and produce hormones that regulate reproductive function and secondary sex characteristics.

Abnormalities in anatomic or physiologic function affect the development and delivery of gametes, and potential fertility.

This book provides a comprehensive review of the anatomy and physiology specific to reproduction, emphasizing developmental and hormonal processes of gamete production, fertilization, implantation, and embryonic development.

This review has been designed to meet the educational needs of physicians and allied health professionals who care for couples experiencing infertility.

By developing a clear understanding of what is normal, you will better understand abnormalities affecting reproduction and the mechanisms behind treatment.

MALE REPRODUCTIVE SYSTEM

OVERVIEW

The male reproductive system is a network of external and internal organs that has three major functions:
- Produce germ cells, called spermatozoa, for sexual reproduction,
- Deliver the male germ cells to the female reproductive tract; and
- Produce hormones that regulate reproductive function and secondary sex characteristics.

Prenatally, the male sex organs are formed under the influence of testosterone secreted from the fetal testes.

Both wolffian and müllerian duct systems are present embryologically.

Wolffian ducts form the male genitalia, and müllerian ducts form the female reproductive tract.

At the 7th week of intrauterine life under the influence of testosterone, wolffian ducts are enhanced.

A substance secreted by the developing gonad (müllerian inhibiting factor) causes the müllerian ducts to regress.

The wolffian ducts develop into the epididymis, vas deferens, ejaculatory duct and seminal vesicles.

In certain structures, male development requires testosterone to be converted to dihydrotestosterone.

With the conversion of testosterone, the urogenital sinus develops into the prostate gland and urethra; the urogenital tubercle becomes the penis and scrotum.

Male gonads are the testes, which produce sperm, fluid, and hormones.

Fluid discharged into the duct system is an exocrine function and hormones represent an endocrine function.

Beginning at puberty, testes produce spermatozoa continuously, not cyclically as in the female.

Sperm produced in the testes is transported through the epididymis, ductus deferens, ejaculatory duct, and urethra.

Concomitantly, the seminal vesicles, prostate gland, and bulbourethral gland produce seminal fluid that accompany and nourish the sperm as it is emitted from the penis during ejaculation and throughout the fertilization process.

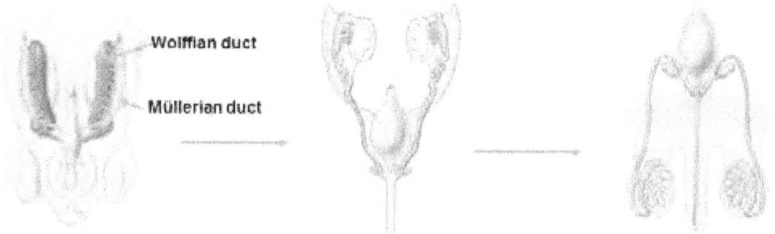

Wolffian Ducts

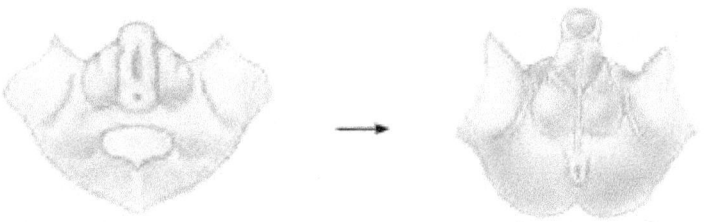

Urogenital Development

♂ - *Overview*

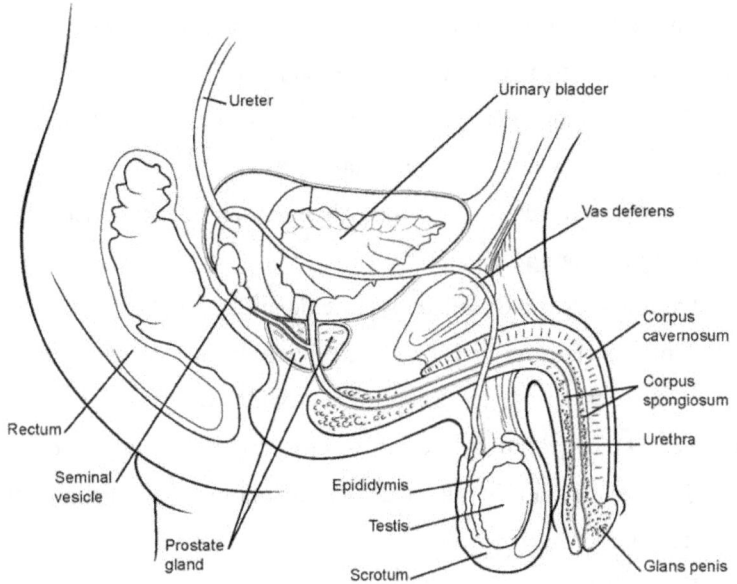

Male Reproductive System

TESTES

The testes are the primary male reproductive organ and are responsible for testosterone and sperm production.

Their development is influenced by the presence of the Y sex chromosome and by maternal hormonal levels.

The testes develop in the fetal abdomen and begin descent during the 7th month of pregnancy.

Failure to descend, called cryptorchidism, results in sterility, which is a lack of spermatozoa, and, frequently, abnormally low testosterone.

Each testis is 4-5 cm long, 2-3 cm wide, weighs 10-14 g and is suspended in the scrotum by the dartos muscle and spermatic cord.

Suspension outside the body cavity permits spermatogenesis to occur at 36°C.

Each testis is covered by the tunica vaginalis testis, tunica albuginea, and tunica vasculosa.

The tunica vaginalis testis is the lower portion of the processus vaginalis and is reflected from the testes on the inner surface of the scrotum, thus forming the visceral and parietal layers.

Beneath the visceral layer of the tunica vaginalis is the tunica albuginea, which forms a dense covering for the testes.

Internal to the tunica albuginea is the tunica vasculosa, containing a plexus of blood vessels and connective tissue.

Bilateral testicular arteries originating from the aorta, just inferior to the renal arteries, provide arterial supply to the testes.

The testicular arteries enter the scrotum in the spermatic cord via the inguinal canal and split into two branches at the posterosuperior border of the testis.

Additionally, the testes receive blood from the cremasteric branch of the inferior epigastric artery and the artery to the ductus deferens.

The pampiniform plexus drains both the testis and epididymis before coalescing to form the testicular vein, usually above the spermatic cord formation at the deep inguinal ring.

Lymphatic drainage via the testicular vessels passes into the abdomen, ending in the lateral aortic and pre-aortic nodes.

The tenth and eleventh thoracic spinal nerves supply the testes via the renal and aortic autonomic plexuses.

Scrotum

The scrotum is a fibromuscular pouch divided by a median septum (raphe) forming 2 compartments, each of which contains a testis, epididymis and part of the spermatic cord.

Layers of the scrotum consist of skin, dartos muscle, external spermatic fascia, cremasteric fascia and internal spermatic fascia, which is in close contact with the parietal layer of the tunica vaginalis.

The skin and dartos layers of the scrotum are supplied by the perineal branch of the internal pudendal artery in addition to the external pudendal branches of the femoral artery.

The layers deep to the dartos muscle are supplied by the cremasteric branch of the inferior epigastric artery.

The veins of the scrotum accompany the arteries, eventually draining into the external pudendal vein and subsequently the greater saphenous vein.

Lymphatic drainage of the skin of the scrotum is by the external pudendal vessels to the medial superficial inguinal lymph nodes .

The scrotum has a rich sensory nerve supply that includes the genital branch of the genitofemoral nerve (anterior and lateral scrotal surfaces), the ilioinguinal nerve (anterior scrotal surface), posterior scrotal branches of the perineal nerve (posterior scrotal surface), and the perineal branch of the posterior femoral cutaneous nerve (inferior scrotal surface).

Microscopic Anatomy

The testes are divided into approximately 400 segments called lobules each of which is occupied by 2-4 seminiferous tubules, which are responsible for producing spermatozoa.

Each testis has 600-1200 seminiferous tubules with a total length of 280-400-m.

At the mediastinum testis, on the posterior border of the testis, the seminiferous tubules empty spermatozoa into the tubuli recti and rete testis, eventually coalescing to form 6-8 efferent ductules draining spermatozoa into the epididymis.

The seminiferous tubule epithelium consists of proliferating spermatogenic cells and the sustentacular Sertoli cells.

Spermatogenic cells are at various stages of spermatogenesis and Sertoli cells are columnar cells that extend from the basement membrane to the lumen of the seminiferous tubule.

Interstitial cells in the testis, including the Leydig cells, constitute 20-30% of the tissue in the gland and are found in between seminiferous tubules.

The washed out cytoplasm of the Leydig cells is due high lipid content in the form of cholesterol for synthesis of testosterone.

Seminiferous Tubules

The seminiferous tubules are the site of spermatogenesis; there are approximately 244 m (800 feet) of seminiferous tubules in each testis.

Each tubule consists of a basement membrane, lined with germ cells that become spermatozoa, and Sertoli cells; these tubules increase in diameter and tortuosity with hormonal changes of puberty.

Cell Types within the Testes

There are three unique cell types within the testes:
− Germ cells, the cells that divide and mature to become sperm;
− Sertoli cells, which provide crucial support for spermatogenesis; and
− Leydig cells that produce the androgenic hormone testosterone, which maintains the reproductive tract and secondary sex characteristics.

All germ cells and Sertoli cells are within the seminiferous tubule, while Leydig cells are outside the tubules.

Sertoli Cells

The Sertoli cells of the testes are joined together by tight junctions that form the blood-testis barrier, which prevents diffusion of plasma constituents into the tubular lumen.

The blood-testis barrier also prevents contact between germ cells and blood, which is important because spermatozoa are antigenic.

Sertoli cells nourish developing sperm, and have a phagocytic function to destroy defective germ cells and engulf extruded cytoplasm from spermatids during remodeling.

Sertoli cells secrete seminiferous tubule fluid, androgen-binding protein and inhibin and activin, which regulate FSH secretion.

Leydig Cells

The interstitial Leydig cells produce and secrete testosterone which is absolutely required for spermatogenesis.

However, FSH greatly enhances spermatogenesis by stimulating the functions of Sertoli cells and increasing mitoses of spermatogonia.

Once mitosis has been initiated in spermatogonia, testosterone alone can maintain spermatogenesis.

Physiology and Function

– Produce germ cells (spermatozoa) for sexual reproduction, and
– Produce testosterone that regulates reproductive function and secondary sex characteristics.

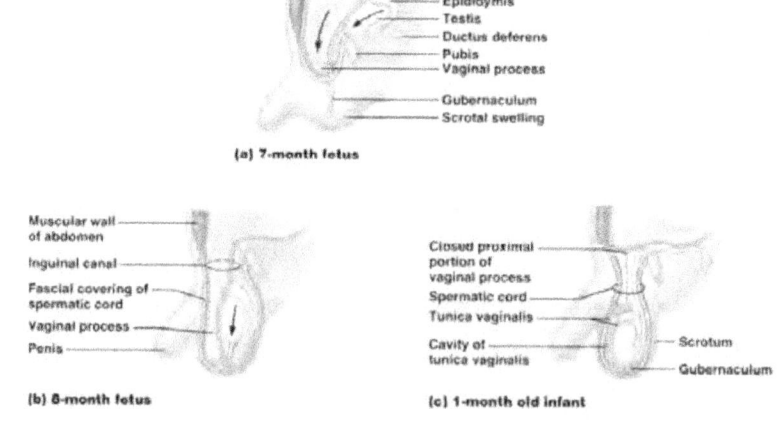

Testicular Descend

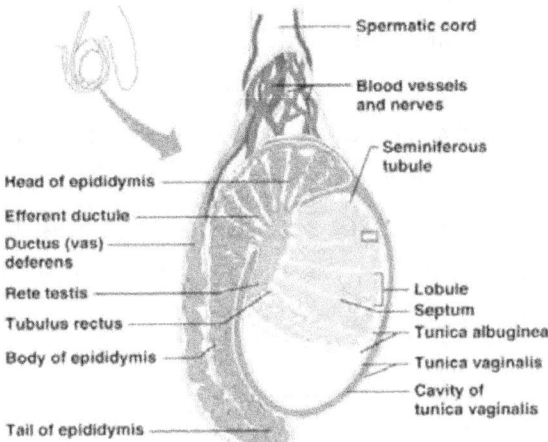

Seminiferous Tubules

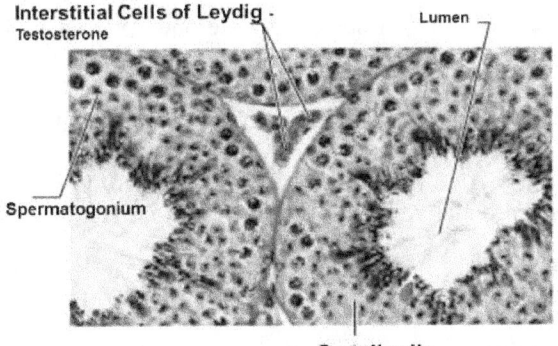

Cell Types within the Testes

HORMONAL CONTROL

Several hormones control testes function:
- Gonadotropin-releasing hormone (GnRH) is secreted by the hypothalamus and stimulates the pituitary to synthesize and release LH and FSH.
- Luteinizing hormone (LH) stimulates Leydig cells to synthesize testosterone.
- Follicle-stimulating hormone (FSH) maintains Sertoli cell function.

Effects of Testosterone

Testosterone has significant reproductive and nonreproductive effects throughout the male life cycle.

Before birth, testosterone masculinizes the reproductive tract and external genitalia and promotes descent of the testes into the scrotum.

For sex-specific tissues, testosterone promotes growth and maturation of the reproductive system at puberty, is essential for spermatogenesis, and maintains the reproductive tract throughout adulthood.

Other reproductive effects include development of the sex drive at puberty and control of gonadotropin hormone secretion; secondary sex characteristics are also testosterone-dependent.

Testosterone induces the male pattern of hair growth (such as the beard), causes the voice to deepen due to thickening of the vocal cords, and promotes muscle growth responsible for the male body configuration.

Nonreproductive actions of testosterone include a protein anabolic effect, promotion of bone growth at puberty and closure of the epiphyseal plates; testosterone also induces aggressive behavior.

Pituitary Feedback

Testosterone provides negative feedback to the pituitary to decrease LH and FSH levels, and to the hypothalamus to decrease GnRH production.

Testosterone only partially decreases FSH production; inhibin, produced by Sertoli cells, is responsible for the remainder of the inhibition of FSH production.

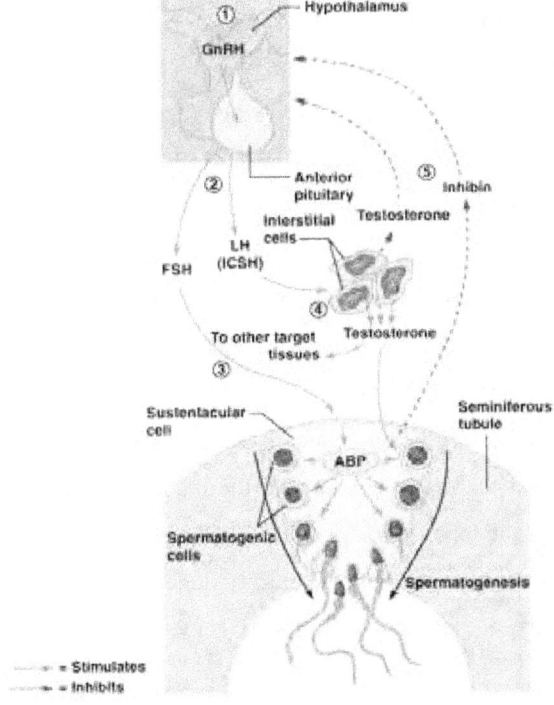

Hormonal Control of Testicular Function

SPERMATOGENESIS

Beginning at puberty, spermatogenesis occurs continuously and repeatedly within folds of the Sertoli cells.

Spermatogonia (the sperm stem cells) lie at the base of the Sertoli cells and proliferate through mitosis to produce daughter cells that enter spermatogenesis.

In the two-step reduction division process of meiosis, spermatocytes and spermatids develop; spermatids are haploid, containing only one copy of each chromosome.

As the germ cells divide and mature, they move away from the base of the tubule toward the apical surface of Sertoli cells.

Spermatogenesis takes 74 days, with several hundred million sperm reaching maturity daily; the process is temperature sensitive, occurring only at temperatures less than or equal to 36°C.

Following meiosis, spermiogenesis is the maturation process in which the round spermatids are transformed into elongated spermatozoa with tails.

The spermatid nucleus condenses and most cytoplasm is lost; the Golgi apparatus moves to one side of the nucleus, forming an acrosome that surrounds the top two thirds of the nucleus (in the head).

Cell microtubules organize into a flagellar apparatus to form the tail for motility, and mitochondria for movement.

Spermiation

Spermiation is the process in which fully developed but non-motile spermatozoa are released from the Sertoli cells and propelled out of the tubules into the collecting tubules, rete testis and then the epididymis.

Mature Sperm

Mature sperm have a head, which consists primarily of the nucleus containing genetic information.

The acrosome is a specialized lysosome, containing about 20 different enzymes, which are needed for penetration of the ovum during fertilization.

The acrosome covers the anterior third of the nucleus in a mature sperm cell.

In the midpiece are mitochondria to provide the energy required for the movement of the tail.

The tail grows out of one of the centrioles; movement results from the sliding of the microtubules.

Normal Sperm Morphology

Normal sperm morphology is defined by multiple parameters:
- The head is oval shaped, 4-5 microns long, 2-3 microns wide, the length-to-width ratio is 1.5 to 1.75, and a well-defined acrosome makes up 40 to 70% of the head area.
- The midpiece is intact and there is no cytoplasmic droplet.
- The tail is 45 microns long, and is not bent or coiled.

Sperm Abnormalities

Sperm abnormalities are scored in four categories:
- For the head, abnormal characteristics include large, small, tapered, pyriform, amorphous, vacuolated, bicephalic, and acrosome defects.
- In the neck and midpiece, a distended or irregular midpiece, thin midpiece (no mitochondria), and bent or absent tail are abnormal.
- Abnormal tails may be short, multiple, hairpin, broken, or coiled.

If there is a cytoplasmic droplet attached at the midpiece, the spermatozoon is considered immature.

Clinical assessment is made on the overall percentage of normal forms; however, prevalent defects should be specifically noted.

Manual Assessment of Sperm Motility

Manual assessment of sperm motility includes determining the percent of sperm that move by counting motile and immotile cells in a counting chamber; 100 minimum are counted.

For qualitative evaluation of forward motion:

0 = immotile,

1 = tail movement with no forward movement of the sperm,

2 = weak forward progression,

3 = active tail movement with good forward progression, and

4 = vigorous tail movement with rapid forward progression.

Supravital staining using eosin to differentiate immotile and dead cells is used when motility is less than 40%.

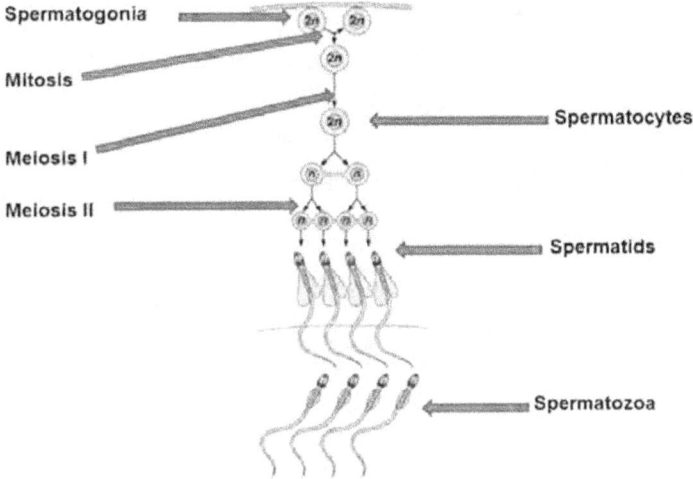

Spermatogenesis

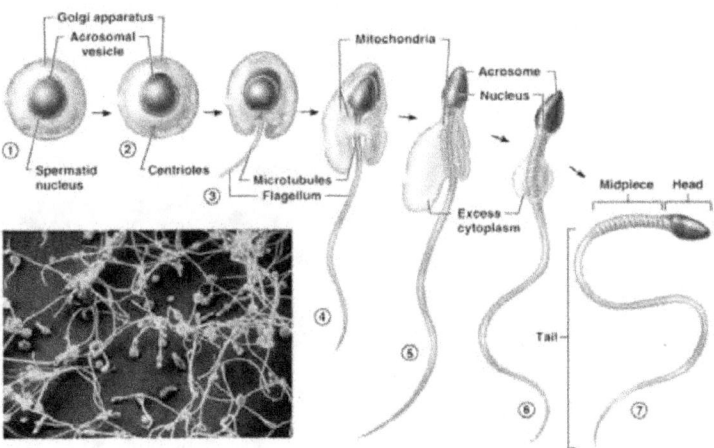

Spermiogenesis

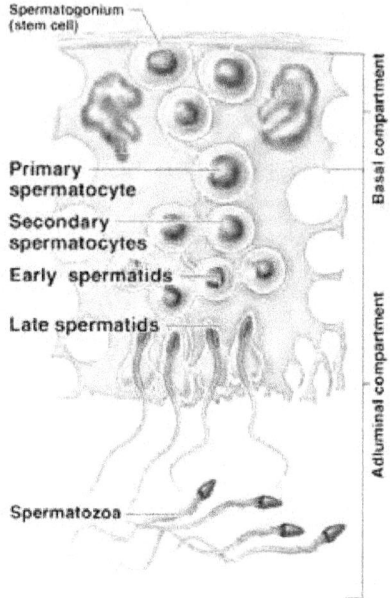

Spermiation

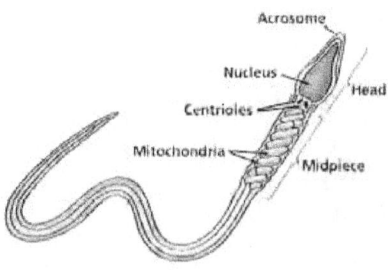

Mature Sperm

DUCT SYSTEM

For each testis there is a duct system; the function of these ducts is testosterone-dependent.

The cells absorb fluid from the testis and remove particulate matter by endocytosis.

The epididymis is where sperm mature, concentrate and are stored for five to six days in this segment of the tract.

The vas deferens is a secondary storage site for spermatozoa; its epithelium has important absorptive and secretory functions.

The other components of the duct system are the ejaculatory duct and the urethra.

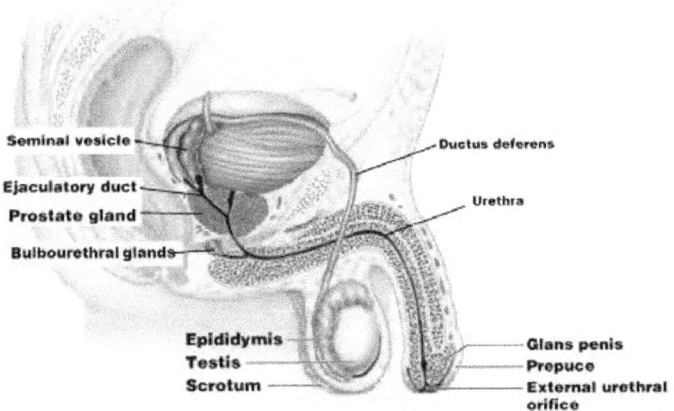

Duct System

EPIDIDYMIS

The epididymis is a C-shaped structure lying intimately along the posterior border of each testis and includes an enlarged head, a body and a tail.

The tunica vaginalis covers the epididymis except at the posterior border.

Vasculature and innervation of the epididymis is the same as for the testes.

Microscopic Anatomy

The main component of the epididymis is a tightly packed, tortuous duct approximately 6-m long and 400-μm in diameter.

The head consists of the most dense pack coils of efferent ductules, which are lined with ciliated columnar epithelium for transport of spermatozoa through the epididymis.

Physiology and Function

The epididymis is the major storage site of spermatozoa, which spend five to six days in this segment of the tract.

When sperm initially enter the epididymis, they are immotile and do not have the capacity to fertilize ova.

Tight junctions between epididymal epithelial cells maintain the blood-testis barrier, which is important for immune protection of sperm.

Epididymal fluid is enriched in potassium relative to semen and rich in glycerophosphorylcholine, a major energy source for spermatozoa.

The epididymis is androgen-dependent, although it responds preferentially to dihydrotestosterone.

The epididymal histology and function change along its length:
- The initial segment connects with the rete testis and has tall columnar cells and a narrow lumen for major fluid absorption.
- In the caput, fluid becomes hyperosmotic and sperm attain motility potential.
- In the corpus, fertilizing potential is achieved with maturation of the sperm plasma membrane and sperm attain the ability to adhere to the zona pellucida of the ovum.
- In the cauda are cuboidal cells with a wide lumen for sperm storage; the luminal fluid becomes acidic as it moves from caput to cauda.

The tall columnar cells of the epididymis secrete ions, nutrients, proteins, and glycoproteins, and they absorb fluid .

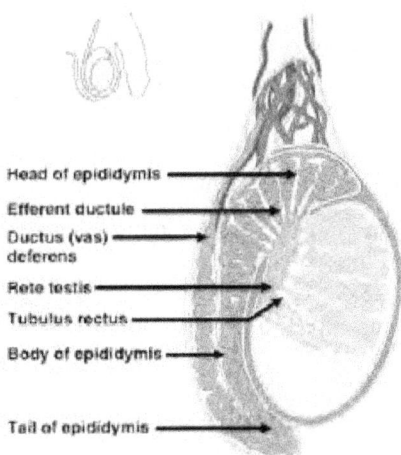

Epididymis

DUCTUS (VAS) DEFERENS

The ductus (vas) deferens is the continuation of the epididymis; it is 30-45-cm long and conveys sperm to the ejaculatory ducts.

The convoluted portion of the ductus deferens becomes straighter (diameter, 2-3-mm) as it travels posterior to the testis and medial to the epididymis.

Subsequently, the ductus ascends on the posterior aspect of the spermatic cord until it reaches the deep inguinal ring, where it participates in the formation of the spermatic cord and loops over the inferior epigastric artery.

At this point, the ductus travels along the lateral pelvic wall, medial to the distal ureter, along the posterior wall of the bladder until it reaches the seminal vesicles dorsal to the prostate.

Each ductus deferens has an artery usually derived from the superior vesical artery (artery to the ductus), with venous drainage to the pelvic venous plexus.

Lymphatic drainage of the ductus deferens is to the external and internal iliac nodes and innervation is mainly sympathetic from the pelvic plexus.

Microscopic Anatomy

The ductus deferens is composed of pseudostratified columnar epithelium including columnar cells and basal cells.

The underlying lamina propria is dense with elastic fibers and the wall of the ductus contains three thick smooth muscle layers.

The outermost layer of adventitia is rich in blood vessels and nerves.

Physiology and Function

In the ductus deferens, there is rapid transport of sperm during ejaculation and slow transport and removal of excess sperm during sexual rest.

The proximal part of the vas is the site of vasectomy for contraception.

The distal part near the prostate, called the ampulla, stores sperm and empties into ejaculatory ducts that traverse the prostate gland to enter the urethra.

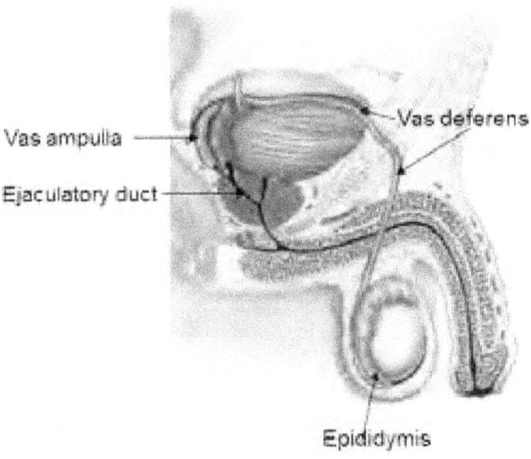

Ductus (Vas) Deferens

Spermatic Cord

The spermatic cord extends from the deep inguinal ring, through the inguinal canal to the testis.

The layers of the spermatic cord include (from outward to inward):
- External spermatic fascia (derived from the deep fascia of the external abdominal oblique muscle),
- Cremasteric fascia (derived from the internal oblique muscle), and
- Internal spermatic fascia (derived from the transversalis fascia).

The structures that form the spermatic cord include:
- The ductus deferens and associated vasculature and nerves (posterior wall of the cord),
- The testicular artery,
- The pampiniform plexus, ultimately forming the testicular vein, and
- The genital branch of the genitofemoral nerve.

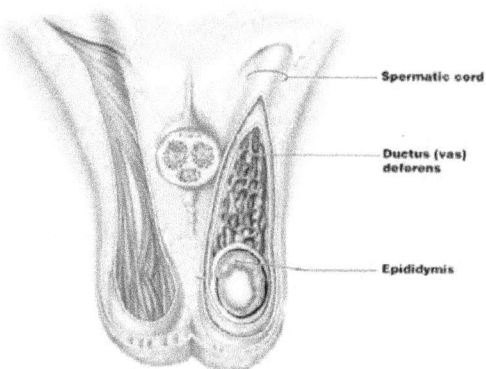

Spermatic cord

EJACULATORY DUCTS

The ejaculatory ducts are 2-cm in length and derived from the union of the seminal vesicle and the ampulla of the vas deferens.

Each duct starts at the base of the prostate and terminates at the seminal colliculus (verumontanum).

The vasculature, innervation, and lymphatics of the ejaculatory ducts are the same as for the ductus deferens.

URETHRA

The urethra stretches from the bladder to the tip of the glans penis, serving as a passage for urine and semen.

The prostatic urethra extends vertically from the bladder neck, through the prostate before becoming the membranous urethra and before penetrating the perineal membrane; of note, the prostatic urethra contains the orifice of the ejaculatory ducts.

As the membranous urethra enters the deep perineal space, the urethra is surrounded by fibers of the external urethral sphincter, eventually entering the bulb of the corpus spongiosum, providing the orifice for the bulbourethral glands and subsequently becoming the penile urethra.

When the urethra reaches the glans penis the diameter diminishes to that of the external ostium, the least dilatable portion of the urethral canal.

Microscopic Anatomy

– The prostatic urethra is lined by transitional epithelium,
– The membranous urethra is lined by stratified columnar epithelium, and
– The penile urethra is initially stratified columnar epithelium and becomes stratified squamous epithelium at the fossa navicularis.

ACCESSORY GLANDS

Accessory glands include the seminal vesicle, prostate gland and bulbourethral glands.

The seminal vesicle provides precursor proteins responsible for semen coagulation, supplies fructose to nourish the ejaculated sperm and secretes prostaglandins that stimulate motility.

The prostate gland secretes proteolytic enzymes to liquefy coagulum after ejaculation, alkaline fluid to neutralize acidic vaginal secretions and the high zinc content is antimicrobial.

The bulbourethral glands, also known as Cowper's glands, secrete mucus for lubrication.

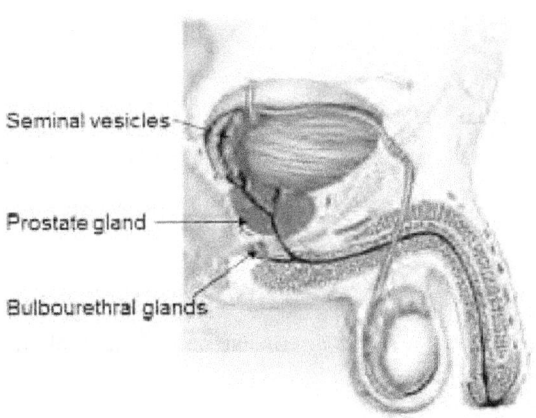

Accessory Glands

SEMINAL VESICLES

The 2 seminal vesicles are located between the bladder and the rectum and measure approximately 5 cm in length.

The anterior surface is in contact with the posterior wall of the bladder and the posterior surface is in contact with rectovesical (Denonvilliers) fascia.

The ampulla of the ductus deferens lies medial to the seminal vesicles and the prostatic venous plexus lies laterally.

Arterial blood supply to the seminal vesicles includes branches from the inferior vesical and middle rectal arteries, while venous and lymphatic drainage accompanies these arteries.

The inferior division of the hypogastric plexus provides innervation to the seminal vesicles.

Microscopic Anatomy

The seminal vesicles are tubulosaccular glands consisting of connective tissue and secretory epithelium projecting into the lumen of the gland.

The epithelium is pseudostratified with basal and columnar cells, while the wall of the vesicle is consistent with a thick wall of smooth muscle that contracts during ejaculation.

Physiology and Function

The seminal vesicles, which are testosterone-dependent, have important secretory function, but they have little storage capacity.

They produce a very alkaline secretion and fibrin, which is responsible for coagulation of semen after ejaculation.

PROSTATE

The prostate gland is an ovoid structure encompassing the proximal portion of the urethra and is approximately 2.5-3.0 cm by 4.0-4.5 cm, normally weighing 20-25 g.

Relations of the prostate gland:
- The base of the prostate is in contact with the bladder,
- The apex is superior to the perineal membrane,
- The anterior border is in contact with the vesicoprostatic plexus,
- The posterior border is separated from the anterior surface of the rectum by the rectovesical (Denonvilliers) fascia, and
- The lateral border is in contact with the levator ani and the prostatic venous plexus.
- Fibers of the external urethral sphincter surround the prostate.

The arterial supply to the prostate gland is derived from the inferior vesical artery and branches of the middle rectal artery.

Venous drainage of the prostate forms the prostatic plexus, which eventually drains into the internal iliac vein and lymphatic drainage flows to the internal iliac nodes.

Innervation is derived from the inferior portion of the hypogastric plexus, primarily to the connective tissue surrounding the gland.

Microscopic Anatomy

The prostate is traditionally divided into three concentric zones:
- The peripheral zone constitutes 70% of the prostate and contains the tubuloalveolar glands of the organ,
- The central zone constitutes 25% and contains submucosal glands and
- The transitional zone constitutes 5% of the prostate.

The tubuloalveolar glands are embedded in a fibrous stroma and open through branching ducts in the prostatic urethra.

The secretory nature of the epithelium is evident as it consists of pseudostratified epithelium containing basal and secretory cells.

Physiology and Function

The prostate gland, which is dihydrotestosterone-dependent, produces a slightly acidic (pH 6.5), colorless, thin secretion, rich in minerals and sodium.

The prostate gland produces the enzyme fibrinolysin, which degrades the fibrin clot in coagulated semen.

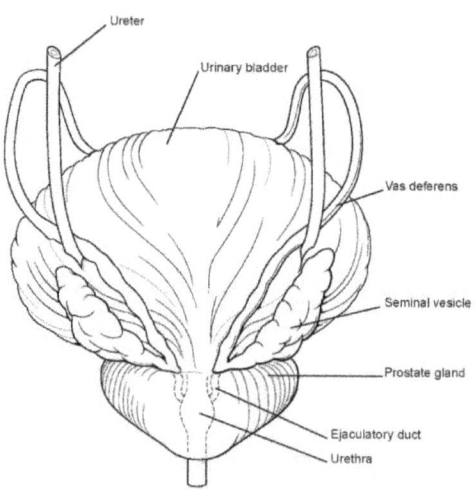

Prostate Gland

BULBOURETHRAL GLANDS

The bilateral bulbourethral glands are 2 cm in diameter and lie lateral to the membranous urethra and are enclosed by the external urethral sphincter.

The excretory duct of the gland penetrates the perineal membrane and opens within the bulbar urethra.

Vasculature, lymphatic drainage, and innervation are generally the same as for the seminal vesicles.

The bulbourethral glands secrete mucus for lubrication during sexual intercourse.

PENIS

The penis is made up of an attached root and a pendulous body; the root consists of two crura and the bulb - 3 bodies of erectile tissue attached to the pubic arch (crura) and perineal membrane (bulb).

Near the border of the pubic sypmphysis the bilateral crura continue as the corpora cavernosa throughout the body of the penis.

The bulb lies between the two crura, narrows anteriorly and continues as the corpus spongiosum.

The corpora cavernosa are enveloped in a thick fibrous tunica albuginea, which is comprised of a longitudinal running superficial fibers and a deep layer of circular oriented fibers.

The corpus spongiosum is penetrated by the urethra as it traverses the body of the penis.

The superficial penile fascia includes loose connective tissue intertwined with dartos muscle fibers.

The deep penile fascia, or Buck's fascia, is a tough fascial layer that encompasses both corpora cavernosa and the corporus spongiosum.

The skin of the penis is thin; the corona of the penis is where the skin folds to become the prepuce (foreskin), enveloping the glans penis.

The vasculature of the penis is extensive; the perineal artery (a branch of the internal pudendal artery) together with the posterior scrotal artery and the inferior rectal artery supply tissues from the bulb of the penis to the anus.

The artery of the bulb of the penis, from the internal pudendal, penetrates the penile bulb and subsequently supplies the corpus spongiosum.

The deep artery of the penis is one of two terminal branches of the internal pudendal artery; it enters the crus of the penis and continues through the length of the bilateral corpus cavernosum.

The other terminal branch of the internal pudendal artery is the dorsal artery of the penis running along the dorsal surface of the penis supplying the penile skin and the glans penis.

The venous drainage of the penis includes the veins draining the corpora cavernosa, which subsequently drains into the circumflex veins.

These veins receive venous blood from the corpus spongiosum on the ventral aspect of the penis and wrap around the penis to drain into the deep dorsal vein.

The superficial dorsal vein drains the penile skin and prepuce before draining via the superficial external pudendal vein into the external pudendal veins.

The deep dorsal vein further drains blood from the glans penis and corpora cavernosa before joining the prostatic venous plexus.

The lymphatic drainage of the penis encompasses three locations:
– The superficial inguinal nodes (penile skin),
– Deep inguinal and external iliac nodes (glans penis), and
– Internal iliac nodes (erectile tissue and urethra).

Sensory innervation to the penile skin is through the dorsal nerve of the penis, one of the terminal branches of the pudendal nerve.

Autonomic innervation includes both sympathetic and parasympathetic aspects to the corpora cavernosum via the cavernous nerves.

The sympathetic fibers originate at the level of T11-T12 and the parasympathetic fibers originate from the pelvic plexus at S2-S4.

Microscopic Anatomy

The erectile bodies of the penis are composed of fibroelastic connective tissue, smooth muscle and a network of vascular sinuses lined with endothelium.

The sinuses are continuous with the arteries that supply them and the veins that drain them.

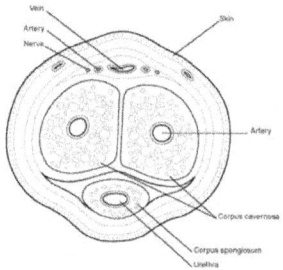

Cross-sectional Anatomy of Penis

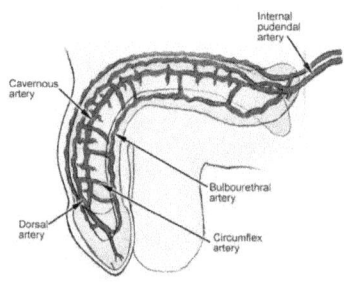

Arterial Supply to Penis

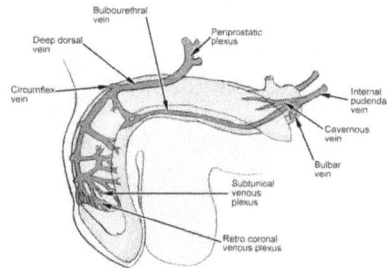

Venous Drainage of Penis

ERECTION AND EJACULATION

In the relaxed state, the central arteries in the cavernosa are constricted, limiting blood inflow; blood flows through sinusoids, and out through veins.

In the aroused state, the central arteries dilate and blood fills the sinusoids to compress the veins, reducing venous outflow and causing an erection.

Emission is a sympathetic and parasympathetic (S2-S4) event causing peristaltic waves up the vas deferens and contractions from the seminal vesicles and prostate gland to expel contents to the prostatic urethra.

Ejaculation is expulsion of the semen in the prostatic urethra distally down the urethra.

Ejaculation occurs by expulsion of the contents of the bulbourethral glands, followed by the fluid from the epididymis and prostate, accounting for about 30% of volume and the highest sperm concentration.

Lastly, the seminal vesicles empty and produce the largest portion of the seminal volume.

Semen is an admixture of sperm cells and secretions from the male accessory sex glands that combine at the time of ejaculation.

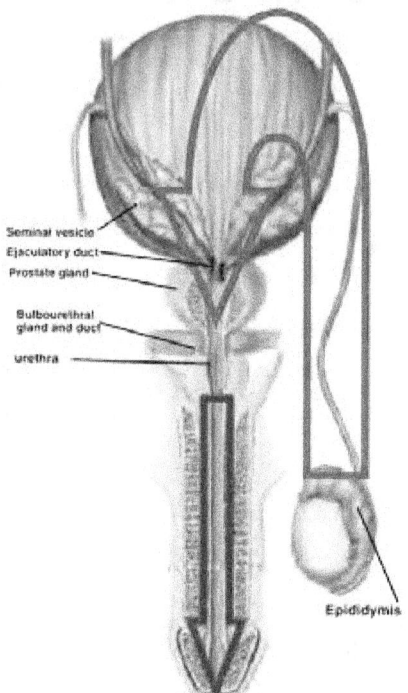

Mechanism of Ejaculation

FEMALE REPRODUCTIVE SYSTEM

OVERVIEW

The female reproductive system is a complicated but fascinating subject.

It has the capability to function intimately with nearly every other body system for the purpose of reproduction.

The female reproductive organs can be subdivided into the internal and external genitalia.

The internal genitalia are those organs that are within the true pelvis: the ovaries, uterine tubes (oviducts or fallopian tubes), uterus, cervix, and vagina.

The external genitalia lie outside the true pelvis: the perineum, mons pubis, clitoris, urethral (urinary) meatus, labia majora and minora, vestibule, greater vestibular (Bartholin) glands, Skene glands, and periurethral area.

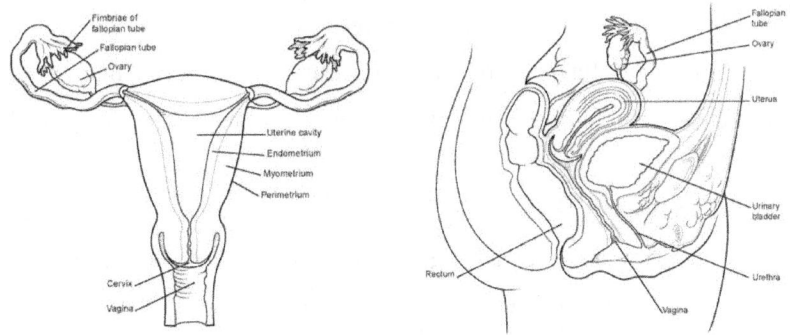

Female Reproductive System

OVARIES

The ovaries are paired organs located on either side of the uterus within the mesovarium portion of the broad ligament below the uterine tubes.

At birth, a female has approximately 1-2 million eggs, but only 300 of these eggs ever mature and are released for the purpose of fertilization.

The ovaries are small and oval-shaped, exhibit a grayish color, and have an uneven surface.

The actual size of an ovary depends on a woman's age and hormonal status; the ovaries are approximately 3-5 cm in length during childbearing years and become much smaller and atrophic once menopause occurs.

A cross-section of the ovary reveals many cystic structures that vary in size representing ovarian follicles at different stages of development and degeneration.

Several ligaments support the ovary:
– The ovarian ligament connects the uterus and ovary.
– The posterior portion of the broad ligament forms the mesovarium, which supports the ovary and houses the vascular supply.
– The suspensory ligament of the ovary (infundibular pelvic ligament), a peritoneal fold overlying the ovarian vessels, attaches the ovary to the pelvic side wall.

Blood supply to the ovary is via the ovarian artery; both right and left ovarian arteries originate directly from the descending aorta at the level of the L2 vertebra, and enter the ovary at the hilum.

The left ovarian vein drains into the left renal vein, and the right ovarian vein empties directly into the inferior vena cava.

Lymphatic drainage of the ovary is primarily to the lateral aortic nodes; however, the iliac nodes may also be involved.

Nerve supply to the ovaries, through the ovarian, hypogastric, and aortic plexuses, run with the vasculature within the suspensory ligament of the ovary entering the ovary at the hilum.

Microscopic Anatomy

The ovaries are covered externally by a layer of simple cuboidal epithelium called germinal (ovarian) epithelium.

Beneath this layer is a dense connective tissue capsule, the tunica albuginea.

The main body of the ovary, or cortex, is divided into an outer cortex and an inner medulla.

The cortex is dense and granular and contains numerous ovarian follicles in various stages of development; each of the follicles contains an oocyte, a female germ cell.

The medulla is loose connective tissue with abundant blood vessels, lymphatic vessels, and nerve fibers.

Physiology and Function

− The ovary cyclically produces gametes; the number of oocytes (germ cells) available is determined during fetal development and continues to decline by either ovulation or atresia until menopause occurs.

− It also cyclically secretes hormones (androgens, estrogens, progestins) that prepare the reproductive tract for oocyte transport, fertilization, implantation and pregnancy, and it controls the hypothalamic-pituitary unit through negative and positive feedback mechanisms.

♀- Ovaries

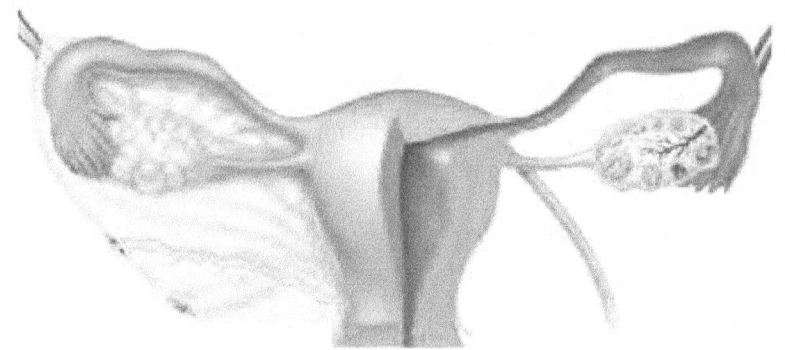

Gross Anatomy of the Ovaries

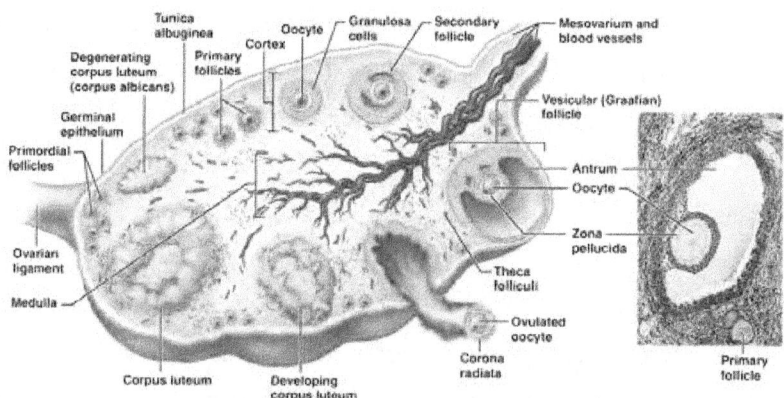

Microscopic Anatomy of the Ovary

HORMONAL CONTROL

There are four major functional compartments involved in reproduction, each has a specific function: the hypothalamus, the pituitary gland and the ovaries, which compose the hypothalamic-pituitary-ovarian (HPO) axis; and the hormonally-responsive functional endometrium lining the uterus.

In the presence of low levels of estrogen, the arcuate nucleus of the hypothalamus releases gonadotropin-releasing hormone.

This hormone signals the anterior pituitary to produce the gonadotropins LH and FSH.

These gonadotropins in turn induce the development and maturation of ovarian follicles that contain the actual oocytes.

During the growth process, the follicles produce increased amounts of estradiol.

This increase in estrogen production develops the endometrium and thins the increasing amounts of cervical mucus.

When the estradiol level reaches an appropriate level, generally when the follicle is mature, the pituitary releases a large amount of LH.

LH surge causes the final maturation of the oocyte and stimulates the event of ovulation.

After the oocyte is released, that is, ovulation occurs, the sac containing the oocyte undergoes metamorphosis with growth of new blood vessels and becomes a functioning gland called the corpus luteum.

The corpus luteum produces progesterone in large amounts and estrogen in smaller amounts.

Progesterone stabilizes the endometrium and thickens the cervical mucus.

The lifespan of the corpus luteum is about 14 days, unless a pregnancy occurs.

If the woman does not conceive in a particular cycle, after 14 days, the corpus luteum stops producing progesterone, the endometrium is no longer stable, and menses begin.

The normal menstrual cycle length is 25 to 35 days; this cyclicity is determined by changing sensitivities of the hypothalamic-pituitary unit to estrogens and progestins.

The HPO axis also involves a negative feedback loop in which gonadal secretions produced in response to pituitary gonadotropins inhibit further secretion of gonadotropins.

The HPO axis in the female also involves a positive feedback loop in which ovarian estrogen produced in response to pituitary FSH enhances pituitary secretion of LH and FSH.

Female Hormones: Production and Action

Functional Compartment	Location	Hormone or Function
- Hypothalamus	- Arcuate nucleus	- GnRH
- Anterior pituitary	- Gonadotropin	- FSH
		- LH
- Ovary	- Follicle	- Estradiol
	- Corpus luteum	- Progesterone
		- Inhibin
		- Activin
		- Anti-Mullerian hormone
- Uterus	- Endometrium	- Proliferative
		- Secretory
		- Menses

Hypothalamus - GnRH

GnRH is synthesized and secreted by neurons in the arcuate nucleus of the hypothalamus and diffuses into the hypothalamic-hypophyseal portal vessels, which transport it to the anterior pituitary gland.

Through pulsatile release, GnRH stimulates the gonadotropes to produce FSH and LH.

The activity of this decapeptide can be modified by changing one or more amino acids; this creates GnRH agonists or antagonists that are often used as adjuncts to infertility and other medical disorders.

Anterior Pituitary - FSH

FSH is a heterodimeric glycoprotein synthesized in gonadotropes in the anterior pituitary.

It has a relatively long half-life in the plasma, normally 3-4 hours; peripheral plasma levels of FSH do not reflect pulsatile GnRH secretion.

FSH stimulates granulosa cells of the ovarian follicle and the luteinized cells of the corpus luteum.

It is considered the critical regulator of follicular development because it is capable of stimulating follicular development by itself.

FSH is suppressed by rising estradiol from the growing follicle; cyclic levels are at their maximum on Day 3 and midcycle surge.

The number of primary follicles which begin to enlarge and respond to FSH is related to the age and total number of oocytes present in the ovary.

Since there is no maturing follicle to suppress FSH, during menopause, FSH is elevated.

Anterior Pituitary - LH

LH is a heterodimeric glycoprotein synthesized in the same gonadotropes in the anterior pituitary as FSH.

LH has a shorter plasma half life (about 20 minutes) than FSH, so peripheral plasma levels do reflect the pronounced pulsatile pattern of GnRH secretion.

LH is secreted in a pulsatile manner:
– In the follicular phase of the female menstrual cycle, the pulse interval is normally 90 min.
– In the luteal phase it is about 2 to 3 hours.

LH stimulates mature granulosa cells of the preovulatory follicle and their successor cells, the luteinized cells of the corpus luteum.

LH is capable of maintaining the lifespan of the corpus luteum beyond the normal luteal phase of the menstrual cycle; however, LH is rapidly degraded when administered by injection.

HCG mimics LH, and can therefore stimulate ovulation and support the luteal phase; hCG has a much longer half life and is slower to degrade when administered by injection.

LH has the following stimulatory effects on ovarian cells:
– Increases availability of free cholesterol.
– Stimulates production of androgens in ovarian theca and interstitial cells by increasing enzymes for androgen biosynthesis.
– Increases production of progesterone and estradiol in the corpus luteum.
– Increases plasminogen activator synthesis and secretion in granulosa cells of the preovulatory follicle.
– Stimulates resumption of meiosis in the oocyte at midcycle.

Ovary – Sex Steroids

Although the ovary secretes many substances steroid hormones including androgens, estrogens and progestins, appear to be among the most important.

Androgens are synthesized in the theca and interstitial cells and are important as substrates for estrogen biosynthesis.

The adrenal glands are the principal source of circulating androgens (dehydroepiandrosterone, androstenedione, and testosterone) in women.

The increase in synthesis of adrenal androgens at puberty (called adrenarche) stimulates the development of axillary, pubic and facial hair.

High levels of androgens suppress progesterone synthesis in granulosa cells.

Although the ovaries and adrenals produce similar quantities of androstenedione and testosterone, most of the ovarian androgens are converted to estrogens in the ovaries and in peripheral tissues.

Most of the testosterone in the plasma of the adult female is formed by peripheral conversion of androstenedione by peripheral 17β-hydroxysteroid dehydrogenase.

Estradiol is considered the most important product of the granulosa cells of the developing follicle; estrone is a less active estrogen than estradiol.

Estradiol concentrations in plasma reach a peak during the late follicular phase, decline after ovulation and then rise again during the luteal phase.

Progesterone is considered the most important product of the corpus luteum.

Ovary – Inhibins and Activins

Inhibin

Inhibin is a heterodimeric glycoprotein consisting of an alpha and a beta subunit and is synthesized by granulosa and luteal cells of the ovary.

FSH stimulates granulosa cells to synthesize and secrete inhibin, so that as follicles enlarge, they produce increasing amounts of the hormone.

Inhibin preferentially inhibits synthesis and secretion of FSH but not LH by pituitary gonadotropes (negative feedback), elimination of inhibin results in a rise in FSH secretion.

Inhibin production is low at the beginning of the menstrual cycle, then increases late in the follicular phase and reaches a peak prior to the preovulatory surge of FSH and LH.

After ovulation, inhibin levels decrease slightly, followed by a final rise in the midluteal phase to a level twice that at midcycle.

As the corpus luteum regresses, inhibin levels decline and FSH levels rise with the beginning of the next menstrual cycle.

Activin

The ovarian granulosa cells secrete activin, a dimeric protein consisting of two of the β subunits of inhibin.

Activin amplifies the effect of FSH on granulosa cells in the ovary and also increases the synthesis of the FSH β subunit in the anterior pituitary.

Activin is synthesized in numerous other tissues, but the role in those tissues is not understood.

Neuroendocrine Control

- Inhibin, acts on the pituitary to suppress the synthesis and release of FSH, but does not impact LH. The effect of inhibin is referred to as negative feedback.
- In the follicular phase, estrogen exerts negative feedback by decreasing the pulse amplitude thereby decreasing FSH and LH pulse amplitude.
- In the luteal phase, progesterone and testosterone decrease GnRH pulse frequency resulting in decreased FSH and LH pulse frequency.
- Testosterone inhibits gonadotropin gene expression in the anterior pituitary; women with elevated serum testosterone levels often do not have normal menstrual cycles.
- GnRH is also inhibited by high concentrations of prolactin; breastfeeding may act as a contraceptive.
- The thyroid can also impact the HPO axis; thyrotropin-releasing hormone (TRH) at high concentrations stimulates the pituitary gland to produce prolactin; patients with hypothyroidism or secondary hyperthyroidism also have decreased gonadotropin secretion.

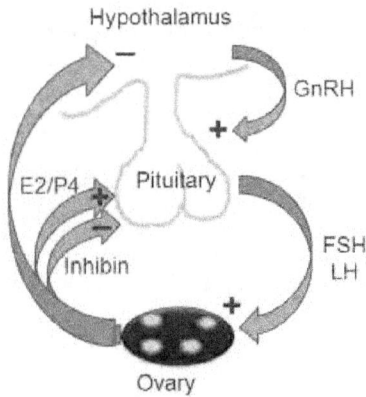

HPO Axis

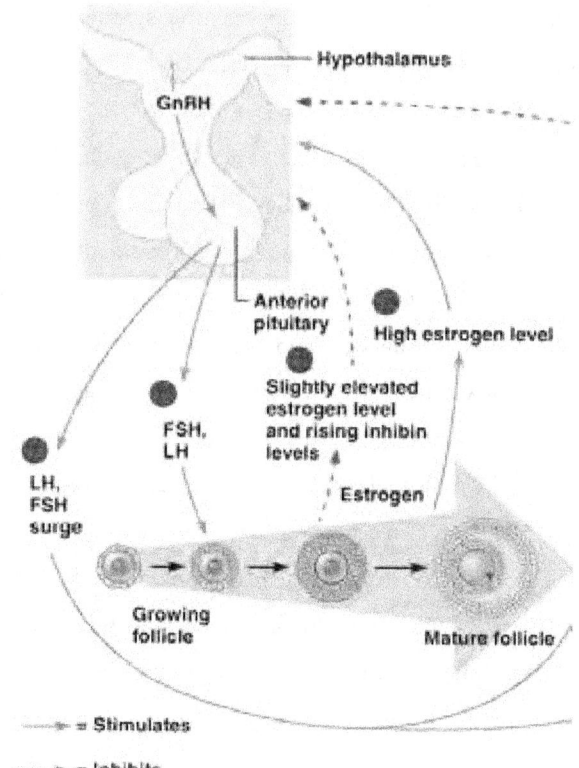

Neuroendocrine Control

OVARIAN CYCLE

The follicle is the basic functional unit of the ovary; each follicle consists of an oocyte surrounded by one or more layers of specialized cells (granulosa, theca) which secrete autocrine, paracrine, and endocrine factors.

The follicle grows under the influence of gonadotropins (FSH, LH) and intraovarian regulators (estradiol, IGF-I, activin).

Development from a primordial follicle to a preovulatory follicle takes three to four menstrual cycles.

Follicular Phase

Primordial Follicle
- Primordial follicles are formed during fetal life and are not believed to require gonadotropins for formation; however, females lacking functional FSH receptors have poorly developed ovaries.
- A primordial follicle consists of an oocyte and a single layer of epithelial cells.
- The oocyte is arrested in the first meiotic prophase.
- During the first cycle of development the oocyte grows to about 100 microns in diameter and the epithelial cells enlarge and become cuboidal granulosa cells; at this point, the oocyte is referred to as the "primary follicle".
- FSH receptors are first detectable on the plasma membrane of granulosa cells.
- The granulosa cells respond to FSH by proliferating faster.

Preantral Follicle

- During the first to second cycles of development, the primary follicle progresses to the preantral stage.
- Oocyte meiosis remains arrested.
- The oocyte completes the first step of meiotic maturation, which includes germinal vesicle breakdown and metaphase I after the mid-cycle LH surge.
- Preantral follicles respond to the midcycle surge of FSH during the second to third cycles of development by growing rapidly; this event is called recruitment.
- All recruited follicles produce sex steroid hormones in amounts proportional to their size and degree of maturation.
- A single follicle, the most mature follicle, becomes dominant.
- The remaining follicles degenerate through a process called atresia.
- The emergence of the single dominant follicle appears to result from the inhibin-induced decline in plasma FSH concentrations.
- Once a dominant follicle is selected, rising serum hormone levels of inhibin and estradiol suppress FSH.
- Local production of estradiol by the dominant follicle amplifies the response to FSH.
- Estradiol synthesis continues to increase exponentially in response to FSH.

Antral Follicle

- Fluid accumulates among the granulosa cells forming a fluid-filled cavity, the antrum.
- After the antrum is formed, the follicle is termed a "secondary follicle".

Preovulatory Follicle
- During the last cycle of development (third or fourth cycle), the dominant follicle attains its maximal size and the theca layer vascularizes; this represents the "Graafian follicle".
- The oocyte (meiosis still arrested) has the capacity to proceed to metaphase II and complete meiotic maturation after fertilization.
- Granulosa cells of immature follicles have few LH receptors so they don't respond to LH at physiological LH concentrations.
- The theca cells (and the interstitial cells) do have LH receptors and they respond to LH.
- One of the actions of FSH on granulosa cells during the follicular phase of the menstrual cycle is to induce LH receptors so that granulosa cells of the preovulatory Graafian follicle become responsive to LH as well as to FSH.
- After the LH/FSH surge prior to ovulation, the granulosa cells initially decrease their LH and FSH receptors and then increase them as the granulosa cells luteinize to become the corpus luteum.

Ovulation Phase
- LH triggers several processes that culminate in ovulation.
- LH causes a resumption of oocyte meiosis, and metaphase I is completed.
- The first polar body is extruded, and meiosis then halts in metaphase II.
- An increase in follicular pressure, combined with LH-activated breakdown of the follicular wall results in follicular rupture.
- The cumulus-oocyte complex is ovulated 34-36 hours after the onset of the LH surge, and the remaining granulosa and theca cells luteinize.

Luteal Phase

- After ovulation the follicular cells luteinize and form the corpus luteum (literally, yellow body).
- They acquire the capacity to secrete progesterone, and lipid droplets accumulate in the cells.
- If the oocyte is fertilized and implants in the endometrium, the corpus luteum remains active and secretes progesterone in large amounts and estradiol in smaller amounts.
- Progesterone from the corpus luteum prepares the endometrium for implantation and maintains the fetal-placental unit during the first half of the first trimester of pregnancy.
- The corpus luteum requires low levels of LH for continued function.
- LH stimulates the production of progesterone and estradiol, and FSH stimulates the production of estradiol only.
- If fertilization and implantation do not occur, the corpus luteum degenerates (called luteolysis), and progesterone declines within 10 days after ovulation.
- Unlike the variable length of the follicular phase of the menstrual cycle, the luteal phase has a lifespan of about 14 days; this lifespan is due to the fairly consistent lifespan of the corpus luteum.
- However, if pregnancy occurs, the corpus luteum is rescued by hCG that is produced by the implanted trophoblasts.
- LH and hCG are similar in structure; hCG may be thought of as long acting LH.
- In clinical situations hCG injections are used to act like LH, particularly to induce ovulation or stimulate luteal progesterone production.

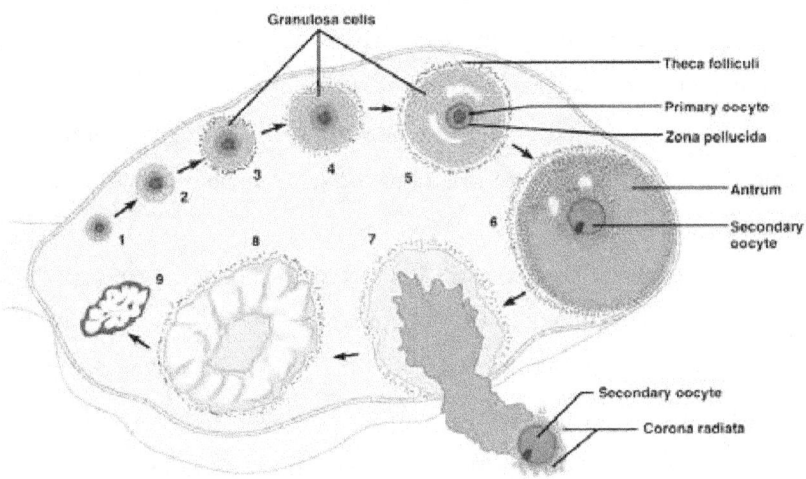

Ovarian Follicular Cycle

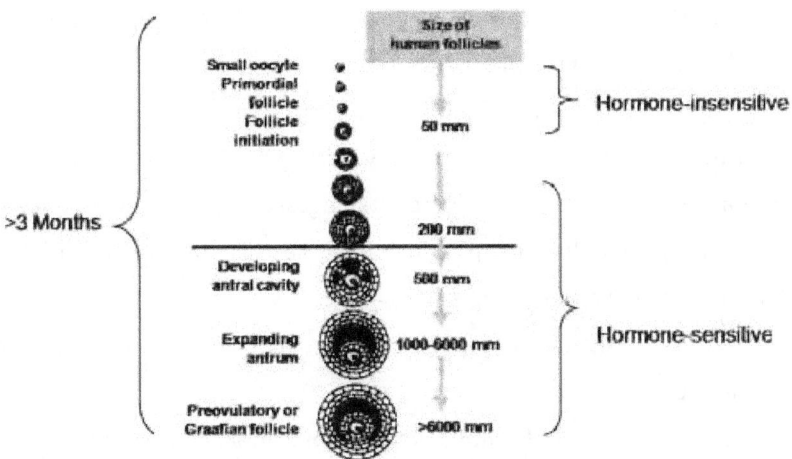

Follicle Development

OOCYTE DEVELOPMENT

The ovaries and germ cells (which develop into oocytes) form during the first few weeks of embryonic life.

These germ cells rapidly divide by a process called mitosis, in which each new daughter cell contains the same number of chromosomes as the parent cell.

During the first trimester of embryonic growth, these preoocyte cells are called oogonium (plural: oogonia).

During the second trimester of life, the 46 chromosomes start to replicate through the process of meiosis but remain within the cell.

At this stage of meiosis, the cell is called a primary oocyte (primitive ovum not yet fully developed).

At this point, further chromosome separation and oocyte development are arrested until after puberty.

These primary oocytes are surrounded by a layer of epithelium that gives rise to the primordial follicles.

About 1700 germ cells are present before migration to the genital ridge begins; however, these multiply during the process of migration, reaching a peak of 7 million oocytes at midgestation.

The primordial germ cells increase in size early in their development and become oogonia.

At midgestation, they begin the first meiotic division, becoming primary oocytes.

This prophase lasts until just before ovulation, which may occur 12 to 40 or more years later.

In this state, they are no longer capable of multiplication and, in fact, steadily decline in number.

About 400 ova are released through the process of ovulation during a woman's lifetime.

The remaining ova undergo atresia (a normal process affecting the primordial ovarian follicles in which death of the ovum results in degeneration) so that, by the time of the menopause, few are present.

The oocyte remains in this stage until it is either eliminated by atresia or succeeds in reaching the maturation stage and resumption of meiosis (reduction division) at the time of ovulation.

Meiosis has two purposes: reduction to the haploid number of chromosomes to one half of the normal, or 23, and recombination of genetic information.

The first meiotic division, which begins during fetal life, is completed prior to ovulation and produces a secondary oocyte containing 23 chromosomes and the first polar body containing 23 chromosomes, each with 2 daughter chromatids.

A polar body is composed of cell division products that result from meiosis.

The second meiotic division, which is initiated after ovulation, is completed at sperm penetration and produces a mature oocyte containing 23 chromosomes and a polar body containing 23 chromosomes, each with a single chromatid.

When the oocyte and sperm combine at fertilization, the full complement of 46 chromosomes is restored and a new life is created; the second polar body will degenerate like the first.

As a result of the combined meiotic processes, a single mature oocyte is produced and 2 or 3 polar bodies degenerate.

This is in contrast to the meiotic process in males where a single precursor cell gives rise to 4 mature sperm.

Oocyte Maturation and Ovulation

— Resumption of meiosis begins within the ovarian follicle in response to the LH surge.
— The granulosa cells, that is, the cumulus oophorus, expands.
— The first polar body is extruded and the oocyte progresses into metaphase of the second meiotic division.
— Meiosis stops in metaphase II until fertilization.

Fertilization

Contractions of the oviductal muscles direct the oocyte into the ampulla of the fallopian tube where it remains for about 3 days while the ampullary-isthmic sphincter remains contracted.

The oocytes remain fertile for only 15-18 hours after ovulation while sperm are motile for 24 hours to several days after ejaculation.

When a sperm encounters the zona pellucida, it undergoes an acrosome reaction; this breaks down the acrosomal membrane.

The sperm head membrane binds to the sperm receptor, which is followed by fusion with the oolemma.

Microvilli on the oocyte surface surround the sperm head and the oocyte undergoes the cortical reaction (release of cortical granules).

The zona pellucida hardens and no other sperm can penetrate the oolemma.

The oocyte nucleus completes maturation to yield the female pronucleus and the second polar body; the sperm nucleus forms the male pronucleus.

The corona radiata is the layer of granulosa cells surrounding the oocyte; the zona pellucida is an extracellular layer of proteins surrounding the oocyte.

Egg activation

The process of egg activation occurs after fertilization, and involves the completion of the second meiotic division and initiation of embryonic development.

Mitosis begins and there are changes in maternal messenger ribonucleic acids and protein synthesis.

Exocytosis of cortical granules blocks polyspermy and cytoskeletal rearrangement occurs.

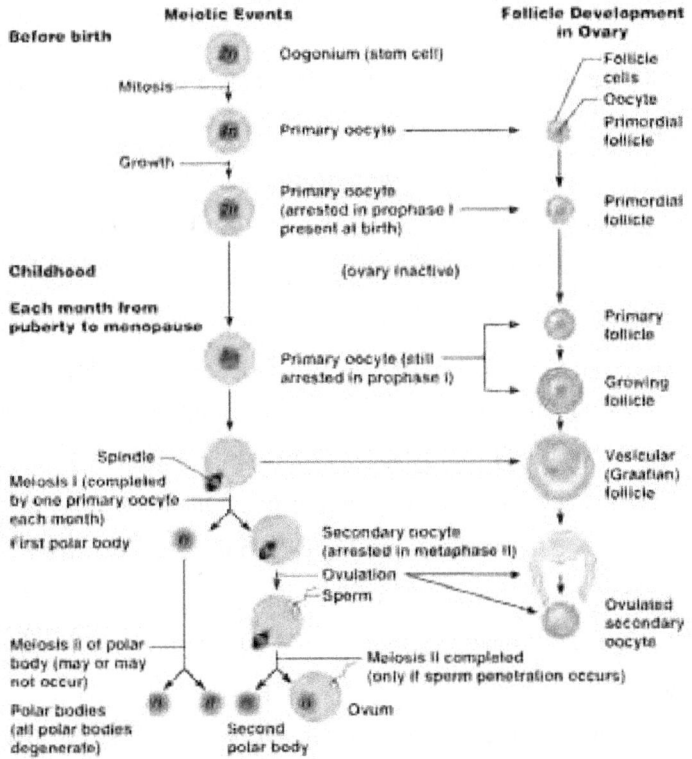

Oocyte Development

UTERINE TUBES

The uterine tubes (also referred to as oviducts or fallopian tubes) are uterine appendages located bilaterally at the superior portion of the cavity.

The uterine tubes exit the uterus through an area known as the cornua and form a connection between the endometrial and peritoneal cavities.

Each tube is approximately 10 cm in length and 1 cm in diameter and is situated within a portion of the broad ligament called the mesosalpinx.

The distal portion of the uterine tube ends in an orientation encircling the ovary.

The uterine tube has 4 parts.
- The first segment, closest to the uterus, is called the isthmus.
- The second segment is the ampulla, which becomes more dilated in diameter and is the typical place of fertilization.
- The final segment, furthest from the uterus, is the infundibulum.
- The infundibulum gives rise to the fimbriae, fingerlike projections that are responsible for catching the egg that is released by the ovary.

The arterial supply to the uterine tubes is from branches of the uterine and ovarian arteries, small vessels that are located within the mesosalpinx.

Lymphatic drainage of the uterine tubes is through the iliac and aortic nodes.

The nerve supply to the uterine tubes is via both sympathetic and parasympathetic fibers; sensory fibers run from thoracic segments 11-12 and lumbar segment 1.

Microscopic Anatomy

The tubal mucosa has many folds, or plicae, which are most evident in the ampulla; a smooth muscular layer surrounds the mucosa.

Within the mucosa of the uterine tubes, 3 different cell types exist:
- Columnar ciliated epithelial cells (25%),
- Secretory cells (60%), and
- Narrow peg cells (< 10%).

Physiology and Function

The released (ovulated) oocyte is guided by waving movements of the infundibulum and fimbriae; muscular peristalsis moves the egg through the fallopian tube.

Fertilization usually occurs in the distal third of the fallopian tube adjacent to ovary (ampulla).

Peristalsis moves the fertilized oocyte through the tubal isthmus and into the uterus for implantation.

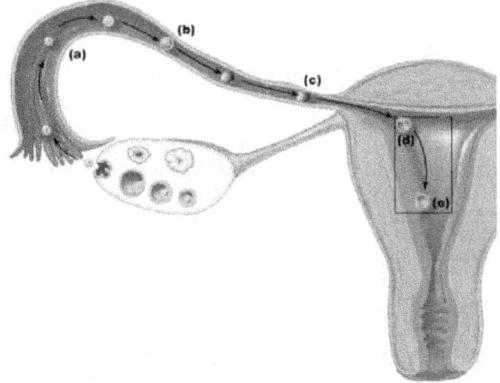

Uterine (Fallopian) Tubes

FERTILIZATION

The fallopian tubes, or oviducts, function as conduits for the oocyte and spermatozoa, and they provide nutrients for the gametes and early embryo, as well as serving as the site of fertilization.

Ciliated cells at the open, fimbriated end (ostium) direct the oocyte into the infundibulum and down through the ampulla.

Estradiol promotes growth, proliferation and ciliogenesis; both estradiol and progesterone increase contractions of the muscular layer to promote transport of the oocyte and fertilized zygote.

The composition of the oviductal fluid is crucial to the survival and development of the zygote; it is tightly regulated by the secretory epithelial cells.

The fluid is enriched in sodium and potassium; oviductal fluid also is enriched in lactic acid and bicarbonate, which are important for cleavage of fertilized eggs or zygotes.

The zygote is kept in the fallopian tube for about three days by the spastic contractions of the estrogen-dominated isthmus; as progesterone increases, muscle tone decreases.

Once the zygote divides it is called an embryo; while still in the fallopian tube, the embryo undergoes cleavage division (1-cell to 8-cell), compaction and blastocyst formation before it reaches the uterus.

The inner cell mass of the embryo becomes the fetus and the outer cells become the placenta and fetal membranes.

Approximately seven days after fertilization, the blastocyst bursts from the zona pellucida, which is called hatching, and implants in the wall of the uterus.

♀- *Uterine Tubes*

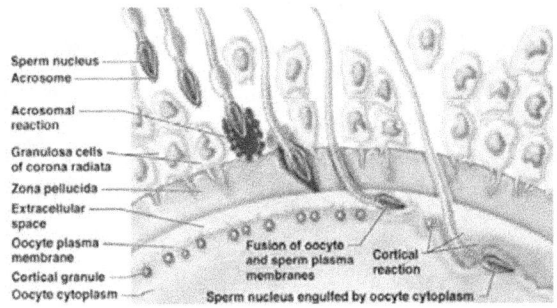

Fertilization

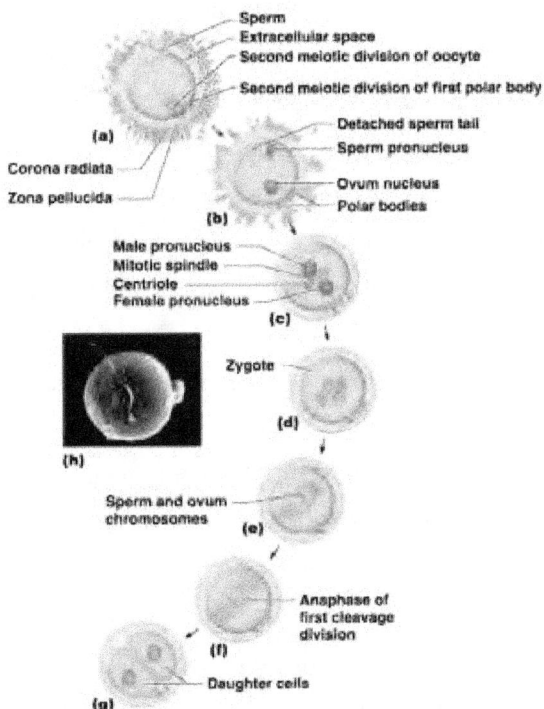

Embryo Cleavage

UTERUS

The uterus is the inverted pear-shaped female reproductive organ that lies in the midline of the body, within the pelvis between the bladder and the rectum.

It is thick-walled and muscular, with a lining that, during reproductive years, changes in response to hormone stimulation throughout a woman's monthly cycle.

The uterus can be divided into 3 parts:
– The most inferior aspect is the cervix, and
– The bulk of the organ is called the body of the uterus (corpus uteri).
– Between these 2 is the isthmus, a short area of constriction.

The body of the uterus is globe-shaped and is typically situated in an anteverted position, at a 90° angle to the vagina.

The upper aspect of the body is dome-shaped and is called the fundus; it is typically the most muscular part of the uterus.

The body of the uterus is responsible for holding a pregnancy, and strong uterine wall contractions help to expel the fetus during labor and delivery.

The average weight of a nonpregnant, nulliparous uterus is approximately 40-50 g.

A multiparous uterus may weigh slightly more than this, with an upper limit of approximately 110 g; a menopausal uterus is small and atrophied and typically weighs much less.

The uterine cavity is flattened and triangular; the uterine tubes enter the cavity bilaterally in the superolateral portion of the cavity.

The uterus is connected to its surrounding structures by a series of ligaments and connective tissue.

The pelvic peritoneum is attached to the body and the cervix as the broad ligament, reflecting onto the bladder, and attaches the uterus to the lateral pelvic side walls.

Within the broad base of the broad ligament, between its anterior and posterior laminae, connective tissue strands associated with the uterine and vaginal vessels help to support the uterus and vagina; together, these strands are referred to as the cardinal ligament.

Rectouterine ligaments, lying within peritoneal folds, stretch posteriorly from the cervix to reach the sacrum.

The round ligaments of the uterus are much denser structures and connect the uterus to the anterolateral abdominal wall at the deep inguinal ring; they lie within the anterior lamina of the broad ligament.

Within the round ligament is the artery of Sampson, a small artery that must be ligated during hysterectomy.

The vasculature of the uterus is derived from the uterine arteries and veins.

The uterine vessels arise from the anterior division of the internal iliac, and branches of the uterine artery anastomose with the ovarian artery along the uterine tube.

Lymphatic drainage is primarily to the lateral aortic, pelvic, and iliac nodes that surround the iliac vessels.

The nerve supply is attained through
– The sympathetic nervous system (by way of the hypogastric and ovarian plexuses) and
– The parasympathetic nervous system (by way of the pelvic splanchnic nerves from the second through fourth sacral nerves).

Microscopic Anatomy

The uterine corpus has 3 layers, from innermost to outermost:
1. The endometrium is composed of of 2 layers:
   - The basal layer lies next to the myometrium and contains stem cells, blood vessels and glands; it builds the functional layer in response to changing levels of estrogens and progesterone produced in the ovary and secreted into the blood stream.
   - The functional layer contains blood vessels and glands.
2. The myometrium is composed of 3 layers of smooth muscle.
3. The serosa is a continuation of the visceral peritoneum.

Physiology and Function

It contains and nourishes the embryo and fetus from the time the fertilized egg is implanted to the time of birth of the fetus.

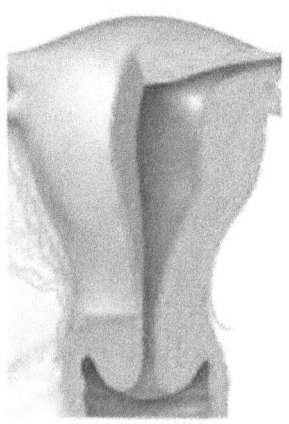

Uterine Cavity

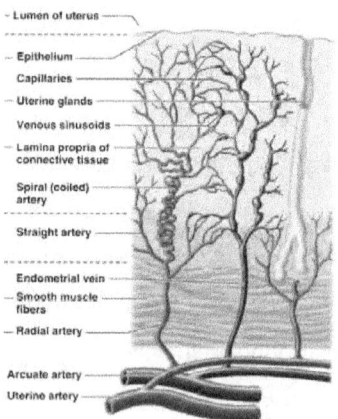

Endometrium

MENSTRUAL CYCLE

Proliferative Phase

The preovulatory follicular phase begins with menses; FSH and LH are released with each GnRH pulse.

Inhibin secretion is low so that FSH, which began to rise late in the luteal phase of the prior cycle, continues to rise; LH levels rise slowly.

Several secondary follicles of different sizes are recruited, and they secrete increasing amounts of estrogen and inhibin.

Estrogen and IGF-I increase the sensitivity of the follicle to FSH, while inhibin blunts the pituitary FSH response to GnRH leading to a decrease in plasma FSH.

The follicle most sensitive to FSH continues to develop and becomes the dominant follicle.

Less developed, that is, less sensitive, follicles undergo degeneration (atresia) because of insufficient FSH.

Estrogen decreases the amplitude of GnRH pulses, as well as increases pituitary sensitivity to GnRH.

Estrogen causes proliferation and vascularization of the endometrium, increases myometrial contractility, and causes the cervical mucus to become clear and thin.

Secretory Phase

When plasma estradiol exceeds 150-200 pg/mL for 36 hours, GnRH triggers a large surge of LH and a small surge of FSH.

The FSH surge recruits new follicles for the next cycle; the LH surge triggers ovulation and luteinization of follicular cells.

The corpus luteum then synthesizes increasing amounts of progesterone, estradiol, and inhibin. FSH and LH are low, but they maintain the corpus luteum.

Progesterone decreases the frequency of GnRH pulses resulting in a decrease in the frequency of LH pulses.

The LH pulse amplitude increases, however, so that plasma LH remains unchanged.

The post-ovulatory rise in progesterone appears to be responsible for the rise in basal body temperature.

Progesterone decreases myometrial excitability and increases endometrial secretory activity.

The luteal phase has a more constant length than the follicular phase.

Menstrual Phase

If implantation of the blastocyst occurs, the lifespan of the corpus luteum is prolonged by hCG, which is produced by the developing embryo.

If implantation does not occur, the corpus luteum regresses; luteal regression begins 14-15 days after ovulation, and progesterone levels decrease to follicular phase levels.

The endometrial lining undergoes ischemic necrosis followed by menses, which is desquamation and bleeding.

Menstruation lasts 3-5 days, and on average, 35 ml of blood + 35 ml serous fluid are lost.

One day before menstruation, when the inhibin levels are low, FSH begins to rise - the proliferative phase is again initiated.

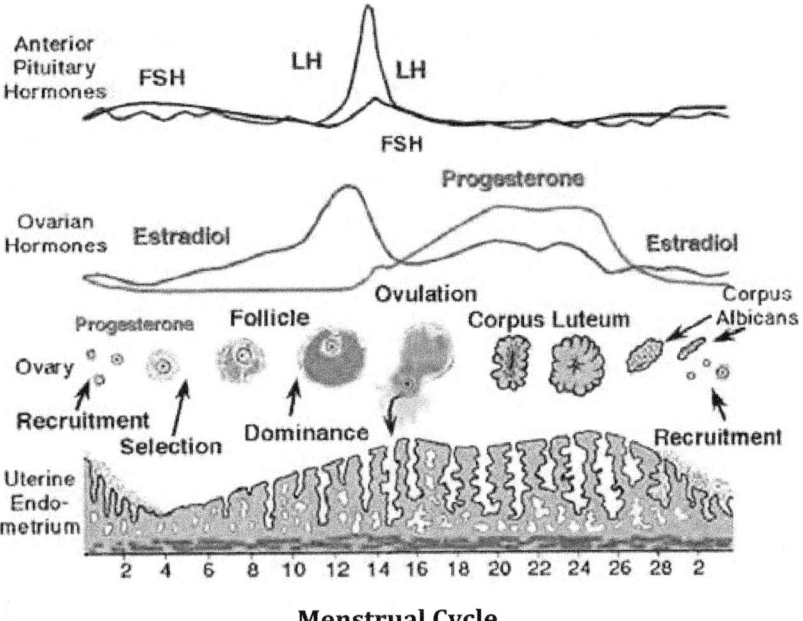

Menstrual Cycle

IMPLANTATION

Approximately seven days after fertilization, the blastocyst bursts from the zona pellucida, which is called hatching, and implants in the wall of the uterus.

Implantation requires prior conditioning of the endometrium by progesterone, which causes the stromal cells to swell and accumulate glycogen, lipids and protein.

The presence of hCG from the blastocyst stimulates the corpus luteum of the maternal ovary to secrete progesterone.

The blastocyst attaches to the wall of the uterine fundus at the embryonic pole.

Trophoblast cells then invade through the endometrial epithelium into the endometrial stroma aided by proteases.

Stromal cells decidualize; a process by which they enlarge and become transcriptionally active, and surround the blastocyst.

The inner cell mass of the embryo becomes the fetus and the outer cells become the placenta and fetal membranes.

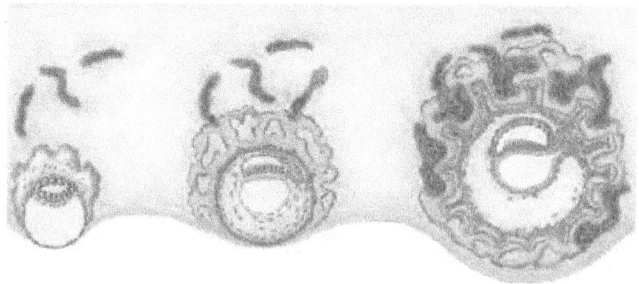

Implantation

EMBRYO DEVELOPMENT

The zygote is kept in the fallopian tube for about three days by the spastic contractions of the estrogen-dominated isthmus; as progesterone increases, muscle tone decreases.

In the fallopian tube, the zygote undergoes cleavage division (1-cell to 8-cell), compaction and blastocyst formation.

The inner cell mass becomes the fetus and the outer cells become the placenta and fetal membranes.

Approximately seven days after fertilization, the blastocyst bursts from the zona pellucida, which is called hatching, and implants in the wall of the uterus, which is called nidation.

Implantation requires prior conditioning of the endometrium by progesterone, which causes the stromal cells to swell and accumulate glycogen, lipids and protein.

The presence of hCG from the blastocyst stimulates the corpus luteum of the maternal ovary to secrete progesterone; anti-progestins such as RU486 can block implantation.

The blastocyst attaches to the wall of the uterine fundus at the embryonic pole.

Trophoblast cells then invade through the endometrial epithelium into the endometrial stroma aided by proteases.

Stromal cells decidualize; a process by which they enlarge and become transcriptionally active, and surround the blastocyst.

Within 11 days of fertilization, the trophoblast forms two layers, the cytotrophoblast and the syncytiotrophoblast, containing lacunae.

The placenta forms a barrier to permit exchange of nutrients, gases and wastes with only slight mixing of fetal blood with maternal blood.

Fetal blood cells can normally be found in the maternal circulation in all cases.

As the lacunae enlarge, the trophoblast forms villi, which consist of a vascularized core of cytotrophoblast covered by syncytiotrophoblast.

The trophoblast erodes the maternal spiral arteries, which then flow directly into the intervillous spaces.

The fully developed placenta consists of the following three layers of membranes:

– Amnion (inner), which is a single layer of ectodermal epithelium completely enclosing the embryo;
– Chorion (outer), which surrounds the amniotic sac and includes the villi and trophoblast; and
– The decidua of the maternal endometrium.

The uterofetoplacental circulation is established by about 6 gestational weeks and is completed by 10 weeks, connecting the maternal decidua through the chorionic villi to the fetus via the umbilical vessels.

Some of the major hallmarks of embryologic development are noted here in developmental weeks.

To correlate with gestational age, adjust by adding 2 weeks to account for time from the last menstrual period to fertilization.

Weeks 3-8

– The period of organogenesis, which is critical for normal development and is the time when most structural birth defects occur.

Week 4

– The neural tube closes.

Week 5
- Limb and facial development begin.
- The embryo appears tightly C-shaped.

Week 6
- Early formation of fingers and toes.
- Brain vesicles are prominent.
- The external ear forms.
- Umbilical herniation begins, caused by swelling from intestinal loops in the umbilical cord and is a normal embryologic event.
- Midgut herniation at this gestational age should not be confused with an omphalocele, which is the abnormal herniation of abdominal organs through an enlarged umbilical ring.

Week 7
- Pigmentation of the retina is seen.
- Fingers and toes separate.
- The upper lip and nipples form.

Week 8
- Limbs are long and bent at the elbows and knees.
- The face is more human-like.
- The tail disappears.

Weeks 11-13
- The bowel returns to the abdominal cavity.
- The long bones and skull ossify.
- The embryo is called a fetus at the 8th gestational week.

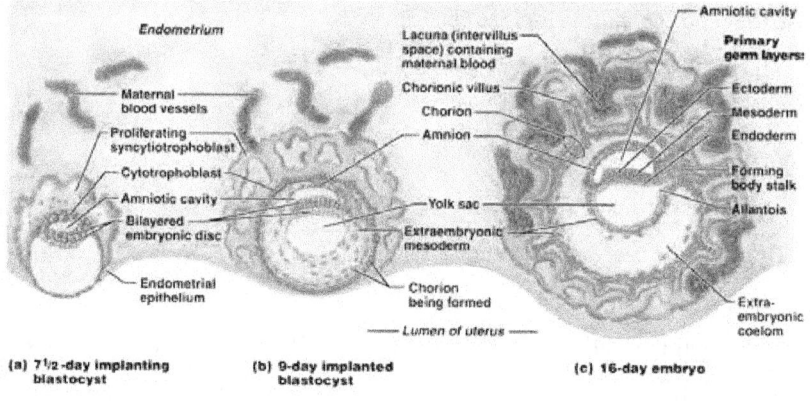

(a) 7½-day implanting blastocyst
(b) 9-day implanted blastocyst
(c) 16-day embryo

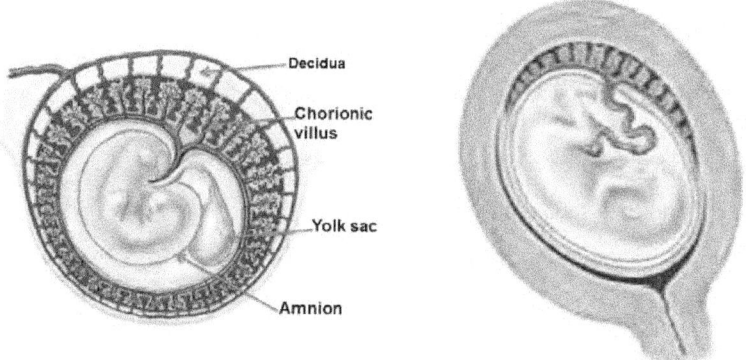

Embryo Development

CERVIX

The cervix is the inferior portion of the uterus, separating the body of the uterus from the vagina; its average length is 3-5 cm.

The cervix is cylindrical in shape, with an endocervical canal located in the midline, allowing passage of semen into the uterus.

The external opening into the vagina is termed the external os; and the internal opening into the endometrial cavity is termed the internal os.

The internal os is the portion of a female cervix that dilates to allow delivery of the fetus during labor.

The vasculature is supplied by descending branches of the uterine artery, which run bilaterally at the 3 o'clock and 9 o'clock position of the cervix.

Lymphatic drainage of the cervix is complex: the obturator, common iliac, internal iliac, external iliac, and visceral parametrial nodes are the main drainage points.

The nerve supply to the cervix is via the parasympathetic nervous system by way of the second through fourth sacral segments; many pain nerve fibers run alongside these parasympathetics.

Microscopic Anatomy

Most of the cervix is composed of collagenous connective tissue, smooth muscle, and mucopolysaccharide ground substance.

The endocervical canal is rich in mucous glands and is primarily columnar epithelium.

The external portion of the cervix that lies within the vagina is composed of stratified squamous epithelium.

The area surrounding the external os is termed the transformation zone, which is the transition point between squamous cells externally and columnar cells of the endocervical canal.

The transformation zone is the area where cervical cell changes (ie, dysplasia) can occur.

Most cell changes are picked up during a Papanicolaou smear, the screening test for cervical cancer.

Physiology and Function

The epithelial lining, of the cervix consists of tall, secretory columnar cells that respond to estradiol by increasing in height and accumulating cervical mucus rich in protein substances.

The mucus functions as a hormone-dependent barrier for sperm to enter the uterus.

At mid-cycle, when estrogen levels are high, mucus is clear, thin, and copious with high elasticity, called spinnbarkeit.

At this point, the cervical mucus is permeable to sperm and when dried, has a characteristic microscopic ferning appearance.

The mucus actually restricts sperm with poor morphology and motility; as a result, only a minority of ejaculated sperm actually enters the cervix.

In response to progesterone production after ovulation, mucus production decreases and it becomes viscous, cloudy, and impermeable to sperm.

VAGINA

The vagina is a 10 to 15 cm musculomembranous tube extending from the uterine cervix internally to the vulva externally.

It is located within the pelvis, anterior to the rectum and posterior to the urinary bladder.

The vagina lies at a 90° angle in relation to the uterus; and is held in place by endopelvic fascia and ligaments

The vagina is lined by rugae, which are situated in folds throughout; these allow easy distention, especially during child bearing.

The structure of the vagina is a network of connective, membranous, and erectile tissues.

The pelvic diaphragm, the sphincter urethrae and transverse peroneus muscles, and the perineal membrane support the vagina.

The sphincter urethrae and the transverse peroneus are innervated by perineal branches of the pudendal nerve.

The pelvic diaphragm primarily refers to the levator ani and the coccygeus and is innervated by branches of sacral nerves S2-S4.

The vascular supply to the vagina is primarily from the vaginal artery, a branch of the anterior division of the internal iliac artery.

Lymphatic drainage of the vagina is generally to:
– The external iliac nodes (upper third of the vagina),
– The common and internal iliac nodes (middle third), and
– The superficial inguinal nodes (lower third).

The nerve supply to the vagina is primarily from the autonomic nervous system.

Sensory fibers to the lower vagina arise from the pudendal nerve, and pain fibers are from sacral nerve roots.

Microscopic Anatomy

The vagina has 3 layers:
- The first layer is the mucosa, the epithelium of which is composed of stratified squamous cells that contain a small amount of keratin; the lamina propria is composed of loose connective tissue that has a vast amount of elastic fibers, giving the vagina its capability to distend.
- The second layer is muscular, mainly smooth muscle.
- The final layer is the adventitia, which is also rich in elastic fibers; a large plexus of blood vessels is also present.

Physiology and Function

It is the receptacle for the penis and sperm during intercourse and the outlet for menstrual flow from the uterus; it is also the birth passageway for the fetus during childbirth.

Vaginal mucosa responds to hormones, especially estrogen, which transforms vaginal epithelial cells from cuboidal to the stratified form for increased resistance to infection and trauma.

EXTERNAL GENITALIA

The vulva, also known as the pudendum, is a term used to describe those external organs that may be visible in the perineal area.

The boundaries include:
– The mons pubis anteriorly,
– The rectum posteriorly, and
– The genitocrural folds (thigh folds) laterally.

The vulva consists of the following organs: mons pubis, labia minora and majora, hymen, clitoris, vestibule, urethra, Skene glands, greater vestibular (Bartholin) glands, and vestibular bulbs.

Mons Pubis

The mons pubis is the rounded portion of the vulva where sexual hair development occurs at the time of puberty.

This area may be described as directly anterosuperior to the pubic symphysis.

Labia Majora

The labia majora are 2 large, longitudinal folds of adipose and fibrous tissue, and have hair follicles.

They extend from the mons anteriorly to the perineal body posteriorly.

Labia Minora

The labia minora are 2 small cutaneous folds that are found between the labia majora and the introitus or vaginal vestibule; anteriorly, they join to form the frenulum of the clitoris.

Clitoris

The clitoris is an erectile structure found beneath the anterior joining of the labia minora.

Its width in an adult female is approximately 1 cm, with an average length of 1.5-2.0 cm.

The clitoris is made up of 2 crura, which attach to the periosteum of the ischiopubic rami.

It is a very sensitive structure, analogous to the male penis; and is innervated by the dorsal nerve of the clitoris, a terminal branch of the pudendal nerve.

Hymen

The hymen is a thin perforated membrane found at the entrance to the vaginal orifice, and varies greatly in shape.

Vestibule

Between the clitoris and the vaginal introitus is a triangular area known as the vestibule, which extends to the posterior fourchette.

The vestibule is where the urethral (urinary) meatus is found, approximately 1 cm anterior to the vaginal orifice, and it also gives rise to the opening of the Skene glands bilaterally.

Urethra

The urethra is composed of membranous connective tissue, and ranges in length from 3.5 to 5.0 cm.

It links the urinary bladder to the vestibule externally, where the urethral (urinary) meatus is found.

Skene and Bartholin Glands

The Skene glands secrete lubrication at the opening of the urethra; the greater vestibular (Bartholin) glands are also responsible for secreting lubrication to the vagina.

Each Bartholin gland is small, similar in shape to a kidney bean, with openings just outside the hymen, bilaterally, at the posterior aspect of the vagina.

Vestibular Bulbs

Finally, the vestibular bulbs are 2 masses of erectile tissue that lie deep to the bulbocavernosus muscles bilaterally.

Microscopic Anatomy

The vulva is predominantly keratinized, stratified squamous epithelium.

The labia majora are composed of both sebaceous and sweat glands; the labia minora are made up of dense connective tissue with erectile tissue and elastic fibers.

The hymen consists of fibrous tissue with a few small blood vessels and is covered by stratified squamous epithelium.

The body of the clitoris is composed of 2 channels of vessels and nerve endings that function as erectile tissue, the corpora cavernosa.

The mucosa of the proximal two-thirds of the urethra is composed of stratified transitional epithelium similar to that of the urinary bladder; the distal one-third is composed of stratified squamous epithelium.

The greater vestibular glands are mostly made up of cuboidal epithelium, with the ducts lined by transitional epithelium.

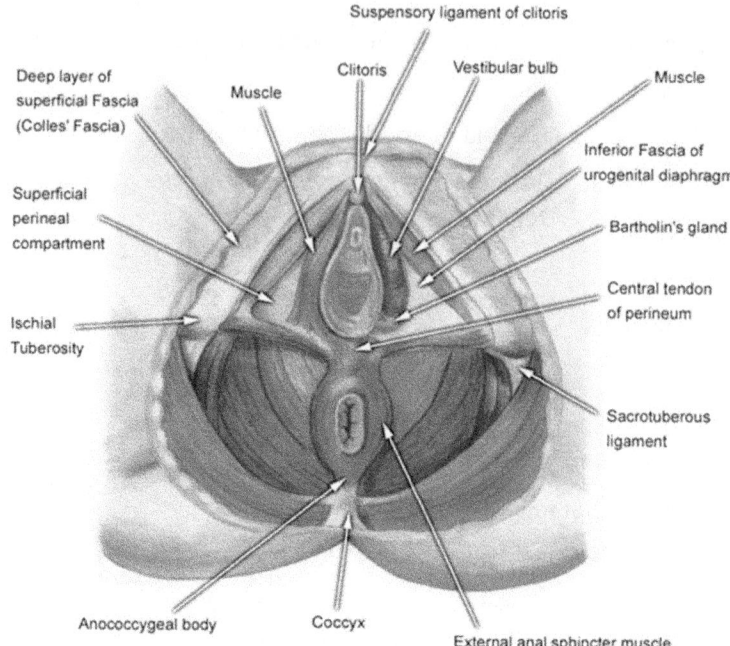

Deep Structures of Female External Genitalia

REFERENCES

- Anson BJ. Morris' Human Anatomy. 12th ed. New York: McGraw-Hill Book Company: A Complete Systemic Treatise; 1966.
- Chung KW. Gross Anatomy. 4th ed. Philadelphia: Lippincott Williams & Wilkins; 2000.
- Drake RL, Vogl AW, Mitchell AWM. Gray's Anatomy for Student's. 2nd ed. Philadelphia: Churchill Livingstone Elsevier; 2010.
- Gillen-water JY, Grayhack JT, Howards SS, et al. Adult and pediatric urology. 4th ed. London: Lippincott. Williams & Wilkins; 2002.
- Gray H. Anatomy, Descriptive and Surgical. The Unabridged Gray's Anatomy. Philadelphia: Running Press; 1999.
- Junqueira LC, Carneiro J, Kelley RO. Basic Histology. 9th ed. Stamford, Connecticut: Appleton & Lange; 1998.
- Katz VL, Lentz GM, Lobo RA, et al. Comprehensive Gynecology. 5th ed. Philadelphia: Mosby Elsevier; 2007.
- Loukas M, Colburn GL, Abrahams P, et al. Gray's Anatomy Review. Philadelphia: Churchill Livingstone Elsevier; 2010.
- Neill J. Knobil and Neill's Physiology of Reproduction. 3rd ed. St. Louis, MO: Elsevier; 2006.
- Ovalle WK, Nahirney PC. Netter's Eseential Histology. Philadelphia: Sauders Elsevier; 2007.
- Sadler T.W. Langman's Medical Embryology. 11th ed. Baltimore, Maryland: Lippincott Williams & Wilkins; 2010.
- Standring S. Gray's Anatomy. 40th ed. Edinburgh: Elsevier Churchill Livingstone; 2008.
- Wein AJ. Campbell-Walsh Urology. 9th ed. Philadelphia: Saunders Elsevier; 2007.

www.ingramcontent.com/pod-product-compliance
Lightning Source LLC
Chambersburg PA
CBHW071755170526
45167CB00003B/1039